Table of Contents

Health Benefits of the MIND Diet 2

Foods to Eat on the MIND Diet 18

Foods to Avoid on the MIND Diet 22

A Sample Meal Plan for One Week 25

How Does the MIND Diet Differ From Other Diet Plans? 30

Will MIND Diet help you lose weight?............... 33

How easy is MIND Diet to follow?...................... 35

Health and nutrition of mind diet 38

Mind diet recipes 46

Possibly Effective For

1) Brain Health

In numerous human and animal studies, foods highlighted in the MIND diet reduced the incidence of Alzheimer's and dementia, and improved memory. This was particularly so in those with healthy brain function or at the very early stages of cognitive decline.

Alzheimer's and Dementia

In a clinical trial of 923 people, modest compliance to the MIND diet for 4.5 years decreased the incidence of Alzheimer's disease by 53% in those over 60 years of age. In comparison, people had to comply very strictly to the Mediterranean or DASH diet to see similar results. The main foods that protect against dementia and Alzheimer's disease are precisely those highlighted in MIND diet (extra virgin olive oil, whole grains, nuts and legumes, and reduced dairy), according to comprehensive reviews on nutrition and brain health, In observational studies of between 2,000 and 10,000 people aged 55 years or older, eating MIND diet foods protected against Alzheimer's and dementia. On the other hand, eating white bread, high-fat dairy products, eggs, meat, fried foods, and sweets was linked to an increased rate of disease. Fish high in omega-3 fatty acids and vitamin D (salmon, herring, mackerel, sardines) should be prioritized. Omega-3s from fish and marine oils were linked to prevention and improvement of Alzheimer's disease. Greatest benefits were seen in people with healthy brain function, those at the earliest disease stages, and in non-carriers of the ApoE4 allele (reviews of observational and clinical studies)

The MIND diet limits alcohol consumption to 1 drink per day, a quantity that protected against Alzheimer's and dementia in observational studies. Inversely, both abstinence and heavier consumption (more than 2 drinks per day) were linked with greater incidence of disease

Memory and Cognition

In a clinical trial of about 500 older people (>70 years of age), the Mediterranean diet enhanced with olive oil or nuts improved cognition more than a low-fat diet. Specifically, polyphenols in olive oil improve learning and memory, according to reviews of human and animal studies, Eating MIND-diet foods improved cognitive function including memory, attention and visual-spatial skills in observational studies of over 23,000 people (aged 58 years or more). Lower intake of vegetables and legumes, specifically, was linked to cognitive decline

2) Inflammation

Chronic inflammation can trigger or worsen many diseases, including Alzheimer's, heart and autoimmune diseases. In some cases, eating mostly MIND-diet-friendly nutrient-dense, plant-based foods and eliminating high-fat and sugary foods can reduce inflammation. Eating MIND diet foods (legumes, whole grains, vegetables, olive oil) for at least 12 weeks lowered markers of inflammation (analysis of 17 clinical trials and about 2,300 people) In a clinical trial with 164 people at high risk for heart disease, a Mediterranean diet that included 1.5 oz of extra virgin olive oil and ¼ cup of nuts per day reduced inflammatory markers by up to 95% compared to low-fat diets in older people (55 − 80 years of age). An observational study of over 24,000 people linked a diet focused on vegetables, olive oil, fruit and fish with lower levels of inflammatory markers (C-reactive protein and white blood cells) in adults.

Omega-3 fatty acids found in fish are well-known anti-inflammatories. They are linked to lower brain inflammation and a slower loss of brain function (reviews of observational, clinical and animal studies).

Olive Oil

Olive oil is the key anti-inflammatory ingredient of the MIND diet. The evidence to back up its benefits is abundant. For example, olive oil reduced inflammation in people over 50 years of age, having a stronger effect in those at higher risk for heart disease (reviews of clinical studies of about 500 people and observational studies of over 40,000 people) Consuming extra virgin olive oil has also been linked to reduced inflammation in autoimmune diseases like rheumatoid arthritis, IBS, amyotrophic lateral sclerosis (ALS), and multiple sclerosis (observational and clinical reviews). Polyphenols from olive oil and red wine reduced inflammation in human cells. Antioxidant polyphenols are possibly the main anti-inflammatory substances in these foods.

3) Cardiovascular Disease

The MIND diet recommends eating plant-based foods high in fiber, complex carbs, vitamins, minerals, healthy fats, and phytochemicals. MIND diet foods reduced the rate of heart disease, deaths from heart disease, total cholesterol, and HDL cholesterol compared to lower-fat diets, according to meta-analyses of observational and clinical trials. Extra virgin olive oil, the primary fat in the MIND diet, helped prevent heart failure, pla1ue build-up in the arteries, irregular heartbeat and heart disease (review of clinical and observational studies). Flavonoids, abundant in berries, were linked to lower LDL cholesterol, triglycerides, lower blood pressure, as well as improved heart health overall (clinical, observational, and animal studies.

4) Diabetes

Eating high amounts of whole grains, fruits and vegetables improved blood sugar control and reduced overall incidence of Type 2 diabetes by about 20% compared to low-fat diets (review of meta-analyses and 5 clinical trials).

One analysis of over 400 observational studies explored the relationship between major food groups in the MIND diet (whole grains, vegetables, nuts, legumes, and fish) and type 2 diabetes. They found that:

10

- Decreasing the consumption of "high risk" foods (red and processed meats, sugary drinks) reduced the incidence of type 2 diabetes threefold;

- Eating optimal amounts of whole grains (2 servings/day), fruits (2-3 servings/day), and vegetables (2-3 servings/day) reduced the incidence of type 2 diabetes by 42%

- Eating 50g/day of whole grains alone reduced the incidence of type 2 diabetes by 25%

In another analysis, most MIND-diet foods were linked with a 20% reduced rate of type 2 diabetes (18 observational studies).

Insufficient Evidence For

The following purported benefits are only supported by limited, low-1uality clinical studies. There is insufficient evidence to support the use of the MIND diet for any of the below-listed uses. Remember to speak with a doctor before starting the MIND diet, and never use it in place of something your doctor recommends or prescribes.

5) **Weight Loss**

The MIND diet is designed for brain health, but the focus on whole, plant-based foods and the reduction of sweets, dairy, fried and fast foods may promote healthy weight loss. The diet is also rich in fiber and low in high-calorie foods.

Plant-based foods (legumes and whole grains) prevented weight gain and obesity better than high-protein, low-fat, and low-glycemic-index diets in observational and clinical studies, Metabolic syndrome is a cluster of conditions that increase the risk of obesity. Eating olive oil, vegetables, whole grains, legumes, and nuts decreased the rate of metabolic syndrome by 35% and reduced the likelihood of weight gain in an observational study of almost 800 young adults.

6) **Depression**

MIND-like diets, high in plant-based foods, reduced the rate of depression in several studies (clinical and observational). The protective effects are likely from eating a combination of these foods, as opposed to taking isolated nutrients. In a clinical trial of 95 postmenopausal women, the DASH diet (one of the parent diets of the MIND diet) for 14 weeks, improved mood and reduced symptoms of depression. In an observational study of almost 16,000 adults, sticking to the Mediterranean diet for 10 years was linked with a decreased incidence of depression. These results were attributed to foods also found in the MIND diet (vegetables, legumes, whole grains, nuts, fish).

7) Parkinson's Disease

In observational studies of over 1.5 million people, diets rich in foods common to the Mediterranean and MIND diets reduced the incidence of Parkinson's disease by 13%.

In another observational study of over 700 people older people, the MIND diet slowed the progression of Parkinson's disease symptoms such as tremors and poor balance.

8) Longevity

In observational studies of over 3,000 people, a MIND-like diet was linked to a longer lifespan in people over 65 years of age. This effect was associated with a slower rate at which the telomeres get shortened, a key indicator of biological aging.

Risks

The Mediterranean and DASH diets are very healthy diets in general . They are extremely high in plant-based foods: fruits, vegetables, plant-based proteins (nuts, seeds, legumes). They are also very high in potassium and magnesium, two electrolytes/minerals we don't typically get enough of through diet. When it comes to eating fish and fish products which the Mediterranean diet recommends more of we need to be careful about some of the potential pollutants and toxins that end up in fish, including mercury and plastic residues. More and more, plastic residues, BPA other persistent pollutants including DDT and mercury are found in fish. So, if you eat fish, it's a good idea to aim low in the food chain and look for sustainably fished (line and pole caught) products. In general though, these are healthy eating patterns that are high in produce, low in saturated fat and good for human health and even the environment. As with any diet, consult with a doctor before starting any new diet plan.

Foods to Eat on the MIND Diet

Here are the 10 foods the MIND diet encourages:

- Green, leafy vegetables: Aim for six or more servings per week. This includes kale, spinach, cooked greens and salads.

- All other vegetables: Try to eat another vegetable in addition to the green leafy vegetables at least once a day. It is best to choose non-starchy vegetables because they have a lot of nutrients with a low number of calories.

- Berries: Eat berries at least twice a week. Although the published research only includes strawberries, you should also consume other berries like blueberries, raspberries and blackberries for their antioxidant benefits.

- Nuts: Try to get five servings of nuts or more each week. The creators of the MIND diet don't specify what kind of nuts to consume, but it is probably best to vary the type of nuts you eat to obtain a variety of nutrients.

- Olive oil: Use olive oil as your main cooking oil.

- Whole grains: Aim for at least three servings daily. Choose whole grains like oatmeal, quinoa, brown rice, whole-wheat pasta and 100% whole-wheat bread.

- Fish: Eat fish at least once a week. It is best to choose fatty fish like salmon, sardines, trout, tuna and mackerel for their high amounts of omega-3 fatty acids.

- Beans: Include beans in at least four meals every week. This includes all beans, lentils and soybeans.

- Poultry: Try to eat chicken or turkey at least twice a week. Note that fried chicken is not encouraged on the MIND diet.

- Wine: Aim for no more than one glass daily. Both red and white wine may benefit the brain. However, much research has focused on the red wine compound resveratrol, which may help protect against Alzheimer's disease.

If you are unable to consume the targeted amount of servings, don't quit the MIND diet altogether. Research has shown that following the MIND diet even a moderate amount is associated with a reduced risk of Alzheimer's disease When you're following the diet, you can eat more than just these foods. However, the more you stick to the diet, the better your results may be. According to research, eating more of the 10 recommended foods and less of the foods to avoid has been associated with a lower risk of Alzheimer's disease, and better brain function over time. The MIND diet encourages the consumption of all kinds of vegetables, berries, nuts, olive oil, whole grains, fish, beans, poultry and a moderate amount of wine.

Foods to Avoid on the MIND Diet

The MIND diet recommends limiting the following five foods:

- Butter and margarine: Try to eat less than 1 tablespoon (about 14 grams) daily. Instead, try using olive oil as your primary cooking fat, and dipping your bread in olive oil with herbs.

- Cheese: The MIND diet recommends limiting your cheese consumption to less than once per week.

- Red meat: Aim for no more than three servings each week. This includes all beef, pork, lamb and products made from these meats.

- Fried food: The MIND diet highly discourages fried food, especially the kind from fast-food restaurants. Limit your consumption to less than once per week.

- Pastries and sweets: This includes most of the processed junk food and desserts you can think of. Ice cream, cookies, brownies, snack cakes, donuts, candy and more. Try to limit these to no more than four times a week.

Researchers encourage limiting your consumption of these foods because they contain saturated fats and trans fats.

Studies have found that trans fats are clearly associated with all sorts of diseases, including heart disease and even Alzheimer's disease. However, the health effects of saturated fat are widely debated in the nutrition world Although the research on saturated fats and heart disease may be inconclusive and highly contested, animal research and observational studies in humans do suggest that consuming saturated fats in excess is associated with poor brain health. The MIND diet encourages limiting your consumption of butter and margarine, cheese, red meat, fried food, pastries and sweets because they contain large amounts of saturated fat and trans fat.

A Sample Meal Plan for One Week

Making meals for the MIND diet doesn't have to be complicated.

Center your meals around the 10 foods and food groups that are encouraged on the diet, and try to stay away from the five foods that need to be limited.

Here's a seven-day meal plan to get you started:

Monday

- Breakfast: Greek yogurt with raspberries, topped with sliced almonds.
- Dinner: Burrito bowl with brown rice, black beans, fajita Lunch: Mediterranean salad with

olive-oil-based dressing, grilled chicken, whole-wheat pita.

vegetables, grilled chicken, salsa and guacamole.

Tuesday

- Breakfast: Wheat toast with almond butter, scrambled eggs.

- Lunch: Grilled chicken sandwich, blackberries, carrots.

- Dinner: Grilled salmon, side salad with olive-oil-based dressing, brown rice.

Wednesday

- Breakfast: Steel-cut oatmeal with strawberries, hard-boiled eggs.

- Lunch: Mexican-style salad with mixed greens, black beans, red onion, corn, grilled chicken and olive-oil-based dressing.

- Dinner: Chicken and vegetable stir-fry, brown rice.

Thursday

- Breakfast: Greek yogurt with peanut butter and banana.

- Lunch: Baked trout, collard greens, black-eyed peas.

- Dinner: Whole-wheat spaghetti with turkey meatballs and marinara sauce, side salad with olive-oil-based dressing.

Friday

- Breakfast: Wheat toast with avocado, omelet with peppers and onions.
- Lunch: Chili made with ground turkey.
- Dinner: Greek-seasoned baked chicken, oven-roasted potatoes, side salad, wheat dinner roll.

Saturday

- Breakfast: Overnight oats with strawberries.

- Lunch: Fish tacos on whole wheat tortillas, brown rice, pinto beans.

- Dinner: Chicken gyro on whole-wheat pita, cucumber and tomato salad.

Sunday

- Breakfast: Spinach frittata, sliced apple and peanut butter.

- Lunch: Tuna salad sandwich on wheat bread, plus carrots and celery with hummus.

- Dinner: Curry chicken, brown rice, lentils.

You can drink a glass of wine with each dinner to satisfy the MIND diet recommendations. Nuts can also make a great snack.

Most salad dressings you find at the store are not made primarily with olive oil, but you can easily make your own salad dressing at home.

To make a simple balsamic vinaigrette, combine three parts extra virgin olive oil with one part balsamic vinegar. Add a little Dijon mustard, salt and pepper, then mix well.

How Does the MIND Diet Differ From Other Diet Plans?

Although the MIND diet doesn't specifically involve exercise, regular physical activity may also help prevent cognitive decline because movement increases blood flow to the brain and helps supply brain cells with nutrients. In fact, regular physical activity can reduce the risk of Alzheimer's disease by up to 50 percent, according to the Alzheimer's Research and Prevention Foundation.Therefore, exercise in conjunction with the MIND diet could provide further protection against memory loss.

The MIND diet is also different from other popular plans because there's no calorie counting and no food groups are eliminated. The paleo diet and ketogenic (or keto) diet are more restrictive than the MIND diet, says Vanessa Rissetto, RD, a nutritionist based in Hoboken, New Jersey. Both of these popular diets minimize the consumption of whole grains, and paleo omits dairy, too. The MIND diet, on the other hand, isn't overly restrictive and emphasizes an increased intake of foods with cognitive benefits. As a result, you're still able to enjoy your favorite meats, sweets, and wines in moderation.

Keep in mind that while this approach is particularly beneficial to those with a higher risk for Alzheimer's disease or dementia, you don't have to be older or have a family history of the disease to benefit from this diet. "Anyone can benefit from the MIND diet due to its overall healthy eating pattern, and there are no negative side effects Because this diet is plant-based and includes many different types of food, it is generally easy to stick with, whether you're preparing meals at home or dining out. However, following this diet may result in a slightly higher grocery bill because of the emphasis on berries and nuts, which can be pricier than some packaged, less-healthy snacks.

Will MIND Diet help you lose weight?

It's possible you will lose weight by following the MIND diet. While the MIND study was not geared toward weight loss, the brain-unhealthy foods frowned upon in MIND such as whole dairy products, pastries, sweets and fried foods are also tied to weight gain. By avoiding these foods, you might take off pounds while staving off dementia. As for the two diets on which MIND was based, some research has linked the Mediterranean diet to weight loss or being less likely to be overweight or obese. As with the DASH diet, you could lose weight on MIND, especially if you design your personal plan with a calorie deficit. However, a study of more than 6,500 obese participants found no effects on body weight or waistline size from following MIND, according to findings published in February 2020 in the Nutrition Journal.

How easy is MIND Diet to follow?

With broad food group recommendations, and "permission" to stick to guidelines loosely, the MIND diet should be easy to follow.

Eating out on the MIND diet is doable. Also, alcohol is allowed in moderation.

Recipes for the MIND diet are increasingly available. Within a few years, several MIND cookbooks have hit the shelves. "Diet for the MIND: The Latest Science on What to Eat to Prevent Alzheimer's and Cognitive Decline," was written by Morris and includes recipes by her daughter, a chef. MIND diet cookbooks by Kristin Diversi, and registered dietitians Julie Andrews and Maggie Moon offer meal plans as well.

There aren't any time-savers with the MIND diet, unless you can enlist help planning, shopping for and preparing meals. Otherwise, you're on your own.

While not specific to the MIND diet, you could probably get and adapt tips from the Oldways website, which is geared toward the Mediterranean diet. Similarly, the National Heart, Lung, and Blood Institute gives advice on healthy eating and is geared toward lowering blood pressure and the DASH diet.

With MIND's emphasis on green leafy veggies, which are rich in fiber, and no calorie-cutting requirement, you can feel as full as you like. Nutrition experts stress the importance of satiety that feeling you've had enough to eat.

If you're used to dishes like veggies cooked in butter, your taste buds will soon adapt to olive-oil flavor. The same goes for foods prepared by frying: You'll get used to baked or grilled versions instead.

Does MIND Diet have any health risks?

The MIND diet doesn't appear to have any health risks. "The DASH and Mediterranean diets have not been shown to have any risks for any disease or condition that I know of," MIND diet developer Morris told U.S. News in 2015. "It's achieved all of the minimum prescriptions of those diets." For example, she said, the MIND diet calls for at least one fish meal per week, as does the DASH diet. But you could eat fish more fre1uently, such as the six weekly servings in the Mediterranean diet. As with any diet, you should check with your doctor if the MIND diet is right for you, particularly if you have any health conditions.

Is MIND Diet a heart-healthy diet?

Both diets on which MIND is based have been found to reduce the risk of high blood pressure, heart attack and stroke.

Rigorous studies show DASH short for Dietary Approaches to Stop Hypertension can lower blood pressure, which if too high can trigger heart disease, heart failure and stroke. DASH has also been shown to increase HDL, or good cholesterol, and decrease LDL, or bad cholesterol, and triglycerides, a fatty substance that in excess has been linked to heart disease. And the Mediterranean diet has been linked to a decreased risk for heart disease, and shown to reduce blood pressure and bad cholesterol.

Can MIND Diet prevent or control diabetes?

The MIND diet may help prevent or control diabetes. Again, limited research on the MIND diet so far is narrowly focused on brain health. That said, its two parent diets may have diabetes-preventive effects. These effects, if supported by further evidence, would also likely be seen for MIND followers. And like the DASH and Mediterranean diets, eating patterns for the MIND diet align with those recommended by the American Diabetes Association.

Prevention: A study published in the journal Diabetologia in August 2013 suggests that people who follow a Mediterranean-style diet have a lower risk of developing Type 2 diabetes compared to others. The study was based on dietary and diabetes data from more than 22,000 people who were followed more than 11 years. Researchers found that those who most closely adhered to a Mediterranean-style diet were 12% less likely to develop diabetes than those who followed it the least.

A study published in January 2014 in the Annals of Internal Medicine focused on more than 3,500 seniors at high risk for heart disease. Seniors who consumed a non-Mediterranean low-fat diet were most likely to develop diabetes. Those who followed a Mediterranean diet supplemented with extra-virgin olive oil were least likely to develop the disease, followed by those on a Mediterranean diet supplemented with nuts. The MIND diet, which singles out olive oil and nuts as brain-healthy food groups, is likely to have similar diabetes-prevention benefits.

Control: A few studies on DASH show favorable results. A small study published in 2011 in Diabetes Care found Type 2 diabetics on DASH reduced their levels of A1C a measure of blood sugar over time and their fasting blood sugar after eight weeks. The MIND diet, which categorizes sweets and pastries as an unhealthy food group, might also help keep blood sugar in check. And similar to DASH and Mediterranean, the MIND diet doesn't involve rigid meal plans or prepackaged foods so you can make sure the foods you eat fit your doctor's advice.

Does MIND Diet allow for restrictions and preferences?

Most people can customize the MIND diet to fit their needs just pick a preference for more information.

Supplement recommended? No supplement is needed with this diet. "It is strictly a food-based diet," Morris says.

Vegetarian or Vegan: You can "absolutely" adapt to the MIND diet as a vegetarian, Morris says. Without any specific guidance or meal plans, however, it'll be up to you to make sure you're getting the nutrients you need without meat and/or dairy. See all plant-based diets »

Gluten-Free: Simply choose gluten-free foods within MIND's guidelines. See all gluten-free diets »

Low-Salt: While MIND doesn't address salt, you could turn to DASH guidelines for staying under 1,500 milligrams of daily sodium. See all low-salt diets »

Kosher: Yes, you could use only kosher ingredients. See all kosher diets »

Halal: It's up to you to ensure your food conforms. While MIND research suggests that a small amount of daily alcohol beats abstaining, you don't have to rigidly stick to the diet guidelines for brain benefits.

See all halal diets »

Is MIND Diet nutritious?

When the MIND diet first appeared in the 2016 Best Diets rankings, experts praised it for presenting new research based on the benefits of a healthy diet pattern for reducing Alzheimer's risk. However, they pointed out that the research was in early stages and longer, more-controlled studies were needed. In April 2016, the National Institute on Aging awarded a $14.5 million grant to the Rush University-led team to launch a randomized, five-year clinical trial of the MIND diet that includes 600 older adults, some who will undergo brain scans to gauge its protective effects.

Mind diet recipes

BRAIN HEALTHY SALAD

INGREDIENTS

For the Red Wine Vinaigrette:

- 1/2 cup extra-virgin olive oil

- 1/4 cup red wine vinegar

- 1/4 cup unsweetened red grape juice

- 1 tablespoon lemon juice

- 1 to 3 teaspoons honey, to taste

- 1/2 teaspoon salt

- Freshly ground black pepper, to taste

For the salad:

- Dark leafy salad greens, such as baby spinach, baby kale, or other superfood greens

- Blueberries

- Walnut pieces, toasted or raw

Preparation

- To prepare the Red Wine Vinaigrette, measure oil, red wine vinegar, grape juice, lemon juice, honey, salt, and pepper into a mason jar. Tightly screw on lid and shake vigorously until everything is thoroughly combined. Alternatively, you may briskly whisk the ingredients together in a medium bowl, or blend them in a blender or mini food processor.

- Fill a bowl or salad plate with a big pile of leafy greens. Sprinkle blueberries and walnuts over the top. Drizzle with dressing and toss to combine.

Crustless Quiche (Frittata)

Ingredients

- 5 eggs

- 1/4 cup milk or substitute

- salt & pepper

- 1 tsp mustard, brown

- 2 tbsp bacon, diced and cooked

- 1/4 cup tomato, diced

- 2-3 scallions, sliced

- 1/2 cup spinach, finely sliced (chiffonade)

- 2 tbsp canola oil, separated

Preparation

- Preheat broiler.

- Use a cast iron skillet or another skillet that can be placed under the broiler.

- Coat skillet with 1 tbsp. oil and heat on stovetop medium-low about 3-5 minutes

3 Bean Turkey Chili

Ingredients

- 1 pound ground turkey

- 2 tbsp olive oil

- 1 medium yellow onion chopped

- 2 cloves garlic minced

- 1/2 cup celery chopped

- 1 large red bell pepper chopped

- 2/3 cup chicken broth

- 3 tbsp chili powder

- 3 whole bay leaves

- 1 15 oz can black beans

- 1 15 oz can pinto beans

- 1 15 oz can red kidney beans

- 1 24 oz can chopped tomatoes canned

Preparation

- Heat olive oil in a large heavy pot on high. Add ground turkey and cook until lightly brown.

- Add chopped onions, celery, garlic, red pepper, and chili powder. Stir to combine and cook for 2-3 minutes.

- Add chicken broth and tomatoes. Bring to a boil then turn down to simmer.

- Drain and rise the kidney beans, pinto beans, and black beans. Add beans to the pot and stir to combine.

- Add bay leaves and let simmer for 20-25 minute

- Serve alone or with optional toppings of sour cream, cilantro, a sprinkle of cheddar cheese or lime wedge.

SUPERFOODS SALAD

INGREDIENTS

- 4 cups Fresh Kale

- 1 1/2 cup Shredded Carrots

- 1 1/2 cup Broccoli Slaw

- 1 1/2 cup Mukimame or deshelled Edamame

- 1 1/2 cup Blueberry

- 64 Cashews 16 per serving

- 1 cup Walnuts 12 to 14 halves per serving

- 1/4 cup hulled Sunflower Seeds

- 1/2 cup Dried Cranberry

LEMON-GINGER VINAIGRETTE

- 1 large Ripe Lemon squeeze as much as you can (if the lemon is smaller, you can use 2)

- 1/4 cup Olive Oil

- 3 tbsp. Apple Cider Vinegar or red wine vinegar

- 1 inch Fresh Ginger grated

- 1 teaspoon minced Garlic

- 1 teaspoon Dried Parsley

- 1/4 teaspoon Chili Powder

- Himalayan Salt to taste

Preparation

- Wash all the vegetables and fruit, then prepare them by slicing, shredding, and grating.

- Slice Kale into bite size pieces, and place in the large bowl.

- Mix everything for lemon-ginger vinaigrette in the glass jar with a fitted lid and season with salt to taste, start with 1/4 teaspoon and taste. Close the lid and shake the jar to combine all the ingredients.

- Pour the vinaigrette over the kale and massage it for about one minute or until the kale is tender. Squeeze the kale using your hands. You will end up with half of the size in the bowl. You got to do this step to make kale tastier.

- Now add all the other ingredients (fruits and vegetables) and lightly toss with the kale.

- Taste and see if you need to add a pinch or two of Salt.

- Serve just a salad immediately or place in the container/jar with a fitted lid and keep in the fridge for up to 2 days.

Brain-Healthy Chocolate Chip Cookies

Ingredients

- 1 ¼ cups almond meal (ground from raw almonds)
- 1 tsp ground flaxseeds
- ¼ cup dairy- and sugar-free dark chocolate (bar or chips), chopped
- ½ cup finely shredded (desiccated) unsweetened coconut
- ½ tsp aluminum-free baking powder
- ¼ tsp sea salt

- ¾ cup pitted dates, soaked in hot water and blended into a paste

- ¼ aquafaba (liquid in a can of chickpeas, low-sodium or no-salt version)

- 2 tbsp safflower oil

- ½ tsp vanilla extract

- 2 tbsp applesauce

Preparation

- In a large mixing bowl, stir together almond meal, ground flaxseeds, dark chocolate chips, coconut, baking powder, and salt.

- Place the dates in hot water, enough to completely submerge them, and soak for 15 minutes. Then drain and place in a small food processor and blend until pureed.

- In a separate bowl, beat aquafaba (using a handheld mixer or whisking vigorously) until light and fluffy with loose peaks. To the aquafaba, add the oil, pureed dates, applesauce, and vanilla. Then add to dry ingredients and mix until just combined. Loosely cover and chill in the refrigerator for at least 30 minutes or overnight.

- Preheat oven to 375°F. Scoop out 1 to 2 tablespoons of dough or use a small melon scoop to form small balls. Press into discs on a parchment-lined baking sheet with a one-inch distance between each cookie to allow for spreading.

- Bake for 13 to 15 minutes or until edges are golden brown. Remove from oven and let cool for 5 to 10 minutes. Transfer to plate with spatula and let cool at room temperature.

Zucchini Recipe

Ingredients

- 1 ½ pounds zucchini, peeled and chopped into bite sized pieces
- 2 garlic cloves, minced
- 2 tbsp olive oil
- ½ lemon, juiced
- 1 ½ tbsp chopped fresh parsley
- salt, black pepper to taste

Preparation

- In a large skillet heat the olive oil over medium heat.

- Add the garlic and cook for 30 seconds or until garlic begins to be fragrant.

- Add the zucchini and saute stirring occasionally until zucchini is tender, about 10- 15 minutes.

- Remove from the heat.

- Drizzle with lemon juice, sprinkle with fresh parsley and season to taste with salt and black pepper.

- Toss to combine and serve.

Mediterranean-Style Scallops Recipe

INGREDIENTS

- Extra virgin olive oil

- 1 shallot, sliced

- ½ red bell pepper, cored, cut into thin strips

- ½ green bell pepper, cored, cut into thin strips

- 4 to 5 garlic cloves, minced

- 10 oz grape tomatoes, halved

- 2 tbsp capers, drained

- Kosher salt

- Black pepper

- ½ tsp oregano

- ½ tsp cumin

- ½ tsp paprika

- 1 lb wild-caught sea scallops (thawed if had been frozen)

- Splash of fresh lemon juice

- Handful fresh chopped parsley for garnish

Preparation

- In a large cast iron skillet, heat 2 to 3 tbsp extra virgin olive oil over medium heat until shimmering but not smoking.

- Add shallots, red bell peppers, and green bell peppers. Raise the heat to medium-high, and cook for about 3 minutes, tossing occasionally.

- Add minced garlic, tomatoes, and capers. Season with just a pinch of kosher salt and black pepper. Add oregano, cumin and paprika. Toss to combine. Cook for another 5 to 7 minutes, stirring occasionally. Keep warm while you work on scallops.

- In a separate skillet, heat another 2 tbsp extra virgin olive oil over medium-high heat. Add scallops and cook for 2 minutes on one side, turn over and cook another 1 to 2 minutes (do not overcook).

- Transfer scallops immediately to the other pan and nestle them in the tomatoes and peppers mixture. Squeeze just a little bit of lemon juice all over. Garnish with parsley.

- Remove from heat and serve immediately over a bed of lemon rice or plain orzo.

Hazelnut-Crusted Halibut with Beet and Spinach Salad

Ingredients

- 1/2 cup (about 2 oz.) whole-wheat pastry flour

- 3 large egg whites, beaten well

- 3/4 cup finely chopped blanched hazelnuts

- 4 (4-oz.) skinless halibut fillets

- 1 1/4 teaspoon kosher salt, divided

- 3/4 teaspoon black pepper, divided

- 3 tablespoons avocado oil or olive oil, divided

- 3 medium-size navel oranges

- 1 1/2 tablespoon balsamic vinegar

- 1 (8.8-oz.) pkg. precooked ready-to-eat beets, cut into wedges (1¾ cups wedges)

- 5 ounces fresh baby spinach

Preparation

- Place flour in a shallow dish. Put egg whites in a second shallow dish. Place hazelnuts in a third shallow dish. Sprinkle fillets with ¾ teaspoon of the salt and ½ teaspoon of the pepper. Working with 1 fillet at a time, dredge in flour, and shake off excess. Dip in egg whites, and then coat in hazelnuts, pressing to adhere.

- Heat 2 tablespoons of the oil in a large nonstick skillet over medium. Add fillets, and cook until nuts are lightly toasted and fillets flake easily with a fork, 4 to 5 minutes per side. Transfer to a plate.

- Using a paring knife, cut peel and pith away from orange flesh. Section oranges, holding fruit over a bowl to collect juices. Reserve segments (you'll have about 1½ cups). Add vinegar and remaining 1 tablespoon oil, ½ teaspoon salt, and ¼ teaspoon pepper to bowl; whisk to combine. Add beets and spinach to bowl; toss lightly to coat. Divide salad and fillets evenly among 4 plates; top with orange segments, and drizzle with any remaining vinaigrette from bowl.

Salmon & Eggs

INGREDIENTS

- 1 shallot or 1/2 red onion

- 1 tablespoon olive oil

- 4 pasture-raised eggs

- 2 teaspoons truffle oil

- 1 teaspoon paprika

- 8 ounces watercress

- 2 tablespoons balsamic or cider vinegar

- 8 ounces smoked salmon

Preparation

- Thinly slice the shallot or red onion.

- Coat a large skillet with half of the olive oil and warm it over medium-high heat. Crack the eggs into the skillet, drizzle with the truffle oil, and sprinkle with paprika. Cook 3 to 4 minutes until the whites are cooked through but the yolks are still soft.

- While the eggs are cooking, prepare the watercress. Coat a separate large skillet with the remaining olive oil. Add the shallot or onion and cook to 2 to 3 minutes until the shallot starts to soften. Add the watercress and cook for 1 minutes until wilted. Sprinkle with the vinegar.

- Divide the mixture among four plates and top each with an egg and 2 ounces of the smoked salmon. Serve immediately.

Grilled Peach Avocado and Arugula Flatbread

Ingredients

- 2 tablespoons extra-virgin olive oil

- 2 tablespoons balsamic vinegar

- 1 teaspoon Dijon mustard

- 1 dash of salt and black pepper

- 1 large ripe peach, washed and sliced

- 2 large whole grain flatbreads or naan bread

- 2 cups arugula, washed and dried

- ½ large ripe avocado, cut into small chunks

- 2 tablespoon grated parmesan cheese

Preparation

- Preheat grill to 400F. In a small bowl, whisk together oil, vinegar, mustard, salt, and pepper.

- Brush vinaigrette dressing onto peach slices. Place them on the heated grill. Pull the top over the grill and allow peaches to cook for 1 to 2 minutes. Flip over and cook for another minute. Remove from grill. Place flatbread on the grill to heat for 30 seconds on each side. Remove from grill. Spread arugula on each flatbread. Gently add grilled peaches and avocado chunks spaced evenly on top of each; sprinkle with parmesan cheese. Drizzle remaining vinaigrette on top and serve.

Sicilian Scrambled Eggs

Ingredients

- 6 organic free-range eggs

- 2 ripe plum tomatoes, diced

- 1/4 cup kalamata olives diced

- 1/4 cup organic grass-fed whole milk

- 1/2 cup feta

- 1 tablespoon extra virgin olive oil

- 2 cloves garlic finely chopped

- 2 cups baby spinach

- 1/2 cup fresh basil

- Sea salt and black pepper

Preparation

- In a medium bowl, whisk together the eggs, tomatoes, olives, milk, and Feta.

- In a large pan, heat the olive oil over medium heat. Add the garlic and cook for 1 minute or until lightly brown. Add the spinach and basil and cook for 1 minute more.

- Add the egg mixture to the pan and toss with a spatula for 2 to 3 minutes. The eggs should be tender but not runny. Add the salt and pepper to taste. Serve immediately.

Meatball Lunch Bowls

Ingredients

Meatballs:

- 500 g ground chicken or turkey (1.1 lb)

- 1 cup grated Parmesan cheese (90 g/ 3.2 oz)

- 1 large egg

- 1 clove garlic, minced

- fresh zest from 1 lemon

- 2 tsp dried Italian herbs or 2 tbsp any chopped

  herbs

- 1/2 tsp sea salt

- 1/4 tsp black pepper

- 2 tbsp ghee or duck fat (30 g/ 1.1 oz)

Lunch Bowls:

- 1 medium cucumber, peeled and sliced (250 g/ 8.8 oz)

- 1 1/4 cup cherry tomatoes or 2-3 regular tomatoes, chopped (188 g/ 6.6 oz)

- 1 large green bell pepper, sliced (164 g/ 5.8)

- 1 small red onion, sliced (60 g/ 2.1 oz)

- 1 large head green lettuce such as butter lettuce or romaine (250 g/ 8.8 oz)

- 3/4 cup homemade Tomato & Basil Dressing (3 tbsp/ 45 ml per serving)

- 5 tsp extra virgin olive oil (25 ml)

Preparation

- In a bowl, mix all of the ingredients for the meatballs: ground chicken, grated Parmesan cheese, egg, minced garlic, lemon zest, herbs, salt and pepper.

- Using your hands, create 25 small meatballs (about 26 g/ 0.9 oz each).

- Heat a large skillet greased with ghee over a high heat. Once hot, reduce to medium-high and add the meatballs. Cook for about 2 minutes or until crisped up and turn on the other side using a fork. Cook for another 2 minutes or until cooked through. When done, set aside.

- Peel and slice the cucumber, halve the tomatoes and slice the green pepper. Peel and slice the onion.

- To assemble the bowls, fold the lettuce leaves inside a 5 Tupperware containers or a bowl. Add the vegetables. If you're making this for meal prep, you can store the vegetables, meatballs and dressing separately in 3 containers and assemble the bowls before serving.

- To serve, add the meatballs (5 into each bowl) and drizzle with the Tomato & Basil Dressing, 3 tablespoons per serving. Drizzle the meatballs with the olive oil. Eat immediately or refrigerate for up to a day. The meatballs can be stored in the fridge for up to 4 days or freezer for up to 3 months.

www.ingramcontent.com/pod-product-compliance
Lightning Source LLC
Chambersburg PA
CBHW072339290526
45794CB00002B/942